53 FACE MASKS

53 FACE MASKS

SKIN GLOWING AND LIGHTENING

ALANI PUBLISHING

LEGAL NOTICE

The author and publisher of this book have strived to be as accurate and complete as possible in the creation of this book, notwithstanding the fact that he does not warrant or represent at any time that the contents within are accurate due to the rapidly changing of nature.

While all attempts have been made to verify information provided in this publication, the author assumes no responsibility for errors, omissions, or contrary interpretation of the subject matter herein. Any perceived slights of specific persons, peoples, or organizations are unintentional.
In practical advice books, like anything else in life, there are no guarantees. Readers are cautioned to rely on their own judgment about their individual circumstances to act accordingly.

This book is not inte̶   use as a source of medical or dermatological advice. All readers are advised to seek services of competent professionals in medical and dermatological fields.

Dedication

Dedicated to the devoted seekers of healthy, vibrant skin, this book is a testament to your commitment to skincare excellence

Contents

Introduction

Mother Nature has bestowed us with lot of natural ingredients that can be used to prepare several skin whitening/lightening home- made facial masks to make your complexion fair, flawless and gorgeously beautiful.

Papaya and Honey Mask

Fresh papaya is not only tasty to eat but is also excellent when it comes to its benefits for the skin. It contains enzymes such as papain and alpha hydroxyl acids that have the ability to dissolve dead cells and remove impurities, which lead to glowing skin. The other ingredient in this mask, honey has antibacterial properties that can protect the skin.

What You Need

- ½ cup fresh papaya pieces
- 1 tea table spoon honey

What You Need To Do

1. Mash the papaya pieces till you get a smooth and thick paste.
2. Add honey to this paste and mix thoroughly.
3. Apply the paste to your face and keep it on for about 20 minutes.
4. Wash your face with warm water.
5. Rinse again with cold water and pat your skin dry.

How Often You Need To Do This: Every night before sleeping.

Best Suited For: Oily skin, normal skin

Caution: Papain can cause allergic reactions in some people. Do not use this remedy if you are allergic to papaya and its products.

Dried Orange Peels and Yogurt

Orange is a commonly found fruit in most households, and it works really well in whitening the skin. It is also rich in vitamin C that acts as a good depigmenting agent.

What You Need

- A few orange peels
- 1 tablet spoon unflavored yogurt

What You Have To Do

1. Dry the orange peels in the sun for two to three days.
2. Once they become almost crisp, grind them till they turn into powder.
3. Mix one table spoon of this powder with the yogurt till you get a smooth paste.
4. Apply the paste to your skin (after cleansing it) and keep it on for about 15-20 minutes.
5. Rinse with warm water.

How Often You Need To Do This: You can do this every alternate day before going to bed.

Best Suited For: All skin types.

Tomato, Yogurt, and Oatmeal Mask

The lycopene in tomatoes, which gives them their characteristic red color, has photo-protective properties that can protect the skin from aging and other age-related issues. Due to the abundance of antioxidants, tomatoes are one of those foods that can make your skin glow. In a Germanic study, the lycopene in tomatoes was also found to protect the skin from cancer. Oatmeal acts as a gentle exfoliant and improves skin health.

What You Need

- 1 tomato
- 1 tea spoon yogurt (fresh and unflavored)
- 1 tea spoon oatmeal

What You Have To Do

1. Cut the tomato in half. Take a tea spoon or two of its juice.
2. Take the oatmeal in a bowl, and add the juice and yogurt to it. Mix well.
3. Apply the mask to cleansed skin and leave it on for about 20 minutes.
4. Rinse with warm water.

How Often You Need To Do This: Preferably two to three times in Week.

Best Suited For: Oily skin, normal skin, combination skin

Milk, Lemon Juice, and Honey Mask

Lemon juice is rich in vitamin C that has been found to have skin lightening effects due to its ability to reduce the production of melanin, the pigment responsible for skin tanning.

What You Need

- 1 table spoon milk
- 1 table spoon lemon juice
- 1 tea spoon honey

What You Have To Do

1. Mix the ingredients in a bowl.
2. Apply the paste to your face (after having cleansed your face) and leave it on for about 20 minutes.
3. Rinse your face with warm water.

How Often You Need To Do This: Do this every alternate night before going to bed.

Best Suited For: All skin types

Caution: If you feel any burning sensation because of the acidity of the lemon juice, take the mask off immediately and rub an ice cube on the area.

Gram Flour and Rose Water (Or Yogurt)

Gram flour has been found to possess antimicrobial properties that can protect the skin from infection. Rosewater can revitalize and moisturize the skin and give it a refreshed look.

Yogurt has been found to improve the brightness of skin. The probiotic bacteria in yogurt have also been found to keep your skin healthy and make it glow.

What You Need

- 2 table spoons gram flour
- 2-3 tea spoons rose water or yogurt

What You Need To Do

1. Mix the ingredients till you get a smooth paste. Use rose water for normal and oily skin and yogurt for dry skin.
2. Apply the mask all over your face and let it stay on for about 20- 30 minutes.
3. Rinse with warm water.

How Often You Need To Do This: You can do this thrice a week before going to bed.

Best Suited For: All skin types

Caution: Make sure you use yogurt instead of rose water if you have dry skin, else this mask will make your skin drier.

Sandalwood Powder

Sandalwood has skin brightening and lightening properties. It inhibits the activity of tyrosinase, thus reducing melanin production. Almond powder and milk provide essential nutrients and cleanse the skin, making your skin healthier and lighter after a few applications.

What You Need

- 1 table spoon sandalwood powder
- 1 table spoon almond powder
- Milk

What You Have To Do

1. Mix the sandalwood and almond powders with enough milk to make a smooth paste.
2. Apply this to clean skin and leave it on for 20 minutes.
3. Wash with lukewarm water. If you feel any dryness after washing, moisturize your skin well.

How Often You Need To Do This: Apply this mask two to three times a week.

Best Suited For: All skin types

Caution: If you have never used sandalwood powder before, do a patch test on a small area on your forearm and observe for 24 hours. If no reaction or irritation develops, you can use this mask on your face.

Pumpkin Mask

Pumpkin is a powerhouse of antioxidants and exfoliating acids. It consists of beta-carotene and vitamins A and C, all of which help in lightening and brightening the skin.

What You Need

- 2 tea spoons pumpkin puree
- ½ tea spoon honey
- ½ tea spoon milk

What You Have To Do

1. For the pumpkin puree, first cut a pumpkin into several pieces. Later, boil them and put them in an immersion blender.
2. Mix two tea spoons of this puree with the honey and milk till you get a uniform paste.
3. Apply this paste to your face and leave it on for about 20 minutes.
4. Rinse with warm water.

How Often You Need To Do This

You can try this before going to bed at night. It is recommended to use this two to three times in a week.

Best Suited For All skin types

Caution: If you suffer from dairy-related allergies, substitute the milk with rose water or aloe vera juice.

Citrus Mask

The citric acid in lemon and grapefruit cleanses and brightens the skin. It acts a natural bleaching agent and also tightens the pores. The proteins found in egg white are found to have antibacterial properties. These can help protect the skin from external infections.

What You Need

- 1 egg white
- 1 tea spoon grapefruit juice
- 1 tea spoon lemon juice
- 2 tea spoons sour cream (should not be fat-free)

What You Have To Do

1. Beat the egg white in a bowl till it is fluffy.
2. Take the sour cream in another bowl and mix the juices of grapefruit and lemon with it.
3. Now add this mixture to the egg white and mix thoroughly.
4. Apply the mixture to your face and leave it on for 15 minutes.
5. Rinse your face with warm water.

How Often You Need To Do This: Thrice a week before going to bed.

Best Suited For: Oily skin, combination skin, normal skin

Caution: People with dry skin can also try out this remedy, but make sure to moisturize your skin well afterwards.

Potato Juice

Potato juice is rich in vitamin C and has antioxidant properties. It is a mild bleaching agent that whitens your skin and also removes dead cells.

What You Have To Do

1. Peel the potato and cut it into inch-sized pieces.
2. Rub the pieces of potato on the areas you want to lighten so that the juice is spread onto your skin.
3. Leave it on for 15-20 minutes and wash with water.
4. You can also grate the potato, squeeze out the juice, and apply it with the help of a cotton pad.

How Often You Need To Do This: Repeat this thrice a week.

Best Suited: For All skin types

Caution: Potato juice can be slightly drying for the skin. Do not forget to use a moisturizer that suits your skin once you rinse the juice off.

Rice Flour and Milk Face Pack

Rice water and rice powder have been used since long by Asian women for softer, lighter, and healthier skin. Studies have proved that rice can protect the skin from UV rays and also possesses anti- aging benefits. Milk soothes the skin and gives it nourishment.

What You Need

- ½ cup raw rice
- 3-4 table spoons milk

What You Have To Do

1. Grind the raw rice to get a fine powder. Mix this powder with the milk to make a paste.
2. Apply this paste onto your skin and leave it on for 20-30 minutes.
3. Wash with warm water.

How Often You Need To Do This Repeat this two to three times a week.

Best Suited For All skin types

Caution: Substitute milk with regular water or rose water if you are allergic to it.

Blueberry Skin Brightening Mask

Blueberries have excellent immunity-boosting properties that can help your skin glow.

What You Need

- A handful of fresh blueberries
- ½ cup plain yogurt

What You Have To Do

1. Crush the blueberries and blend the paste with the yogurt.
2. Mix well and apply the mask to your face.
3. Leave it on for 15 minutes, and then wash off with warm water.

How Often You Need To Do This: Do this twice a week before going to bed.

Best Suited For: All skin types

Caution: Check for allergic reactions if you are unsure if blueberries will suit your skin or not.

Masoor (red lentil) daal and rose petals fairness face pack

Ingredients

Raw milk, 2 table spoons of masoor daal, 2 table spoons of almond oil and 3 table spoons of fresh rose petals

Procedure

Soak up masoor daal in raw milk for 2 hours and then grind this to make a smooth paste. To this, add fresh rose petals, almond oil and then apply on your perfectly cleansed face. Leave this preparation on for 20 minutes and then wash off after with cold water.

Benefits: This fairness facial mask removes tan and gives a rosy bloom to your face. If used daily for 7 days, your will see a pinkish glow on your face with visibly skin lightening effects.

Chirongi and banana face mask for improving your skin tone

Ingredients

- 2 table spoons of chirongi,
- 2 table spoons of almond oil. One ripe banana,
- Raw milk

Procedure

Soak up chirongi in milk, grind chirongi and full ripe banana together to get a fine lump-free paste and then add 2 table spoons of almond oil. Massage this mixture onto your face using upward strokes and neck for 5 minutes and then keep this mask on face for 20 minutes. Afterwards, wash off with lukewarm water to complete the process.

Benefits: This face mask gives a healthy boost of moisture to your dry and dull skin. With regular use of this beauty tip, your skin will restore its lost charm and sheen. Use this daily for one week and you will notice a positive change in your complexion. Best suited for dry skin.

Sunflower oil and milk face packfor lightening your skin tone

Ingredients

- 2 table spoons of sunflower oil,
- 2 table spoons of curd,
- 3 table spoon of milk powder

Procedure

Mix 3 table spoons of milk powder with 2 table spoons of sunflower oil and 2 table spoons of curd and use this mix to massage your face and neck in upward motion and massage your skin for ten minutes. Next take stream while the fairness mask is on your face to remove all sorts of dirt, pollutants and clear melanin deposit too.

Benefits: This face pack deep cleanses your skin and make it flawlessly clear. Benefits of this homemade facial equals to a parlor clean up. Use this beauty tip twice a week.

Almonds, barley flour and raw milk, essential oil fair skin face pack

Ingredients

- 6 almonds,

- 2 table spoons of barley flour,

- 4 table spoons of raw milk and Few drops of essential oil

Procedure

Soak up almonds in milk and grind them to make a fine paste and then add barley flour and raw milk in this solution and then add few drops of essential oil. Clean your face with cotton swab using rose water and then apply this face mask and leave it on your skin for 10 minutes.

Benefits: This fairness tip makes your skin baby soft and fairer with every usage. Moreover, this home remedy removes fine lines and early signs of wrinkles to reveal a youthful skin.

Sunflower oil, rose water, honey, multani mitti and curd for fairness

Ingredients

- 2 table spoons of sunflower oil
- 3 table spoons of multani mitti,
- One table spoon of honey,
- One table spoon of curd

Procedure

Combine all ingredients to prepare a paste and apply the resultant mix on your face.

Benefits: This beauty tip makes your skin fair and irresistibly smooth On the top of it, this facial mask removes dark spots and brown spots on the face too.

Multani mitti (fuller's earth), honey, papaya tomato, milk skin bleaching mask

Ingredients

- 2 table spoons of multani mitti,
- 2 table spoons of papaya pulp,
- Few table spoons of milk,
- One table spoon of honey,
- 2 table spoons of tomato pulp

Procedure

Wash your face using a mild cleanser and pat dry with a towel. Next, massage coconut oil all over your face and neck for 5- 10 minutes. Next, mix honey, papaya, multani mitti, tomato and honey and slather your face with this home-made facial mask. Let it dry for 20 minutes and wash off with cold water.

Benefits: This facial mask tightens your skin and removes all sorts of impurities to reveal a fresher and fairer skin.

Rose petals, milk cream, urad daal (split black gram) paste, saffron and milk face pack for white skin

Ingredients

- 1 table spoon of split black gram (urad daal),
- 2 table spoon of milk cream,
- 4 strands of saffron,
- Few table spoons of rose petals,
- 4 table spoons of milk

Procedure

Soak up urad daal and saffron, almonds in milk for 2 hours and grind them to get a fine paste. To this, add two table spoons of milk cream. Smear the preparation on your face and wash off after 20 minutes.

Benefits: This natural remedy is helpful in making your cheeks pinkish and rosy. Use this face mask continuously for 10 day and you will surely become fairer and smoother.

Aloe vera and rose water fair skin and anti-tan home remedy

Ingredients

- 2 table spoons of aloe vera gel and

- Rose water

Procedure

Extract the gel out of freshly plucked aloe vera plant and mix this with rose water and apply on all exposed parts of your body.

Benefits: Aloe vera and rose water face mask soother and relaxes sunburnt skin and removes tanning as well as makes your skin fair and spotless.

Curd and Multani mitti, orange juiceface pack to bleach your facial skin

Ingredients

- 2 table spoons of thick curd,
- 3 table spoons of multani mitti and
- 4 table spoons of orange juice

Procedure

Mix all these skin bleaching agents together and apply on your skin for 20 minutes.

Benefits: Orange lightens the facial hair, multani mitti tightens the skin pores and lactic acid present in curd whitens and evens out your skin. Use this beauty tip daily to see fast results.

Split Bengal gram (chana daal), curd and lemon juice mint powder, neem mask for lighter skin tone

Ingredients

2 table spoons of chana daal (split Bengal gram), 2 table spoons of curd,

One table spoon of mint and Neem paste each, juice of a lemon

Procedure

Soak up chana daal in water for 2 hours and to this, add mint paste, lemon juice, neem paste, curd and apply on the skin.

Benefits: Chana daal bleaches your skin and mint and neem have anti-bacterial properties whereas curd removes blemishes and lemon juice lightens acne scars. All these skin whitening agents in this home remedy work in synergy to give you a fairer and blemishes - free skin naturally.

Marigold flower, almond powder and barley flower and curd to make your skin lighter

Ingredients

- 2 table spoons of crushed marigold flowers,
- 2 table spoons of almond powder,
- One table spoon of barley flower and
- Some rose water

Procedure

Combine 3 table spoons of marigold flowers with 2 table spoons of almonds powder and one table spoon of barley flour and rose water. Apply this mask on your skin for 20 minutes.

Benefits: Marigold has anti-septic properties and barley cools the skin whereas almond powder moisturizes your skin. All these natural ingredients work wonders in making your skin lighter and bright.

Turmeric and curd face pack for spotlessly fair complexion

Ingredients

- 2 pinches turmeric,
- 2 table spoons of curd

Procedure

Mix 2 table spoons of curd with 2 pinches of turmeric. Slather on your face for ten minutes.

Benefits: Turmeric not only lightens skin but also heals pimples and rashes and curd removes pigmentation marks to make your skin lighter and brighter. This fairness tip is recommended for all skin types.

Multani mitti, rose water and honey skin whitening mask

Ingredients

> 3 table spoons of multani mitti

> 5 table spoons of rose water and

> 2 table spoons of honey

Procedure

Mix all ingredients together and apply on your face for 20 minutes.

Benefits: This face mask is best for teenager with acne and pimple prone skin. This face mask makes your complexion fairer as well as gets you rid of pimples, acne and acne scars too.

Orange juice, sugar and honey natural bleach for your skin

Ingredients

- 2 table spoons of orange juice,
- 1 table spoon of sugar,
- One table spoon of honey

Procedure

Mix one table spoon of sugar to 4 table spoons of orange juice and blend till sugar dissolves completely and then add one table spoon of honey. Apply the resultant solution on your face, neck and any part of body you wish to lighten. Wash off after 15 minutes.

Benefits: This recipe is natural bleach for your skin minus any chemicals. This mask nourishes your skin to make it velvety and very glowing.

Walnut and milk cream, honey and turmeric powder face exfoliating mask to get instant whitening effects

Ingredients

- 2 table spoons of walnut powder,
- 2 table spoons of milk cream
- One table spoon of honey and
- Half table spoon of turmeric powder

Procedure

Mix all aforementioned ingredients well and whip up a facial mask to get fair skin instantly and apply on your skin. Leave it on for 15 minutes and scrubs off gently to remove dead skin cells and impurities.

Benefits: Rich in vitamin E, walnut nurtures the skin and sloughs off dead skin cells and milk cream makes your skin supple smooth and honey restores the health of skin and turmeric heals the skin. All these magical ingredients mixed together whiten your skin just after one application. Use this fairness scrub thrice a week to get amazing fairness and radiance on your skin naturally at no great cost.

Jasmine flower, curd camphor face whitening mask

Ingredients

- 2 table spoons of jasmine flower paste,
- 2 table spoons of sandalwood,
- 2 pinches of camphor

Procedure

Mix all ingredients together and apply on your face for 20 minutes.

Benefits: The powders of these natural ingredients make your skin gorgeously fair and drool worthy. Moreover, this flower face mask has anti-ageing qualities to make your skin youthful.

By now, you are aware of the best fairness face packs you can prepare at your home. Now incorporate these facial masks into your beauty routine and get set to flaunt a fair, smooth and glowing skin naturally.

Turmeric Face Mask

Things Needed

- Gram flour (Available in Indian stores)
- Organic turmeric powder
- Organic honey
- Milk
- Lemon

Method

You'll need one teaspoon each of gram flour, turmeric powder, milk, and honey. Squeeze a¼ piece of lemon into the mixture. Mix your ingredients gently.

If you have dry skin, add one tsp of yogurt and a few drops of olive oil as well. Wear a band to avoid getting your hair onto your face. Also, wear an old tee shirt while applying the mask. Rub the leftover lemon onto your face. It is always better to exfoliate your skin before you apply any mask and lemon is a natural exfoliator.

Smear the mask with a brush. Spread the mask to the neck as well. Let the mask dry for 20-30 minutes and then wash your face with lukewarm water. When you clean, make sure to gently rub the skin, and exfoliate to get the best results. You can remove the light yellow turmeric stain on your face with a face wash. You can also remove it using the makeup remover, but anyway it will go off in 2 hours' time.

Benefits: Turmeric is rich in antioxidants which fights free radicals and reduces the signs of aging and corrects an uneven skin tone.

Turmeric regulates the production of sebum an oily substance produced by the sebaceous glands. Hence it is perfect for oily skin. It has antibacterial properties and combats acne. It fights dark circles and enhances your skin tone.

Clay Mask

The cosmetic clay conditions and nourishes your skin and removes dead cells, impurities and extra oils from your skin's surface. There are different types of clay such as the Bentonite clay, French green clay, Rhassoul clay and Red clay.

Ingredients

- One tsp Bentonite clay
- 1-2 tsp of distilled water or rose water

Method:

Mix one teaspoon of clay with one teaspoon of distilled water or rose water. It is important that you use non-metal spoon and bowl while mixing Bentonite clay. Apply this mask on the face and allow it to dry for 15-20 minutes.

Rinse the mask with lukewarm water and splash with cold water to close your skin pores. You can add oats, honey, essential oils, orange peel and herbs like chamomile and lavender to the clay mixture to enhance your beauty glow.

Benefits: Bentonite clay helps the cells to get more oxygen. When your facial cells receive more oxygen, it brightens your skin. The clay mask unclogs the skin pores and shrinks them. Bentonite clay reduces the overproduction of sebum and removes the toxins. It helps in exfoliation, makes your skin softer, and reduces the appearance of wrinkles.

Papaya Cucumber Banana Face Mask

Things Needed

- ¼ cup ripe papaya

- ½ banana

- ¼ cucumber

Method: Peel and blend all the ingredients in a blender until you get a smooth puree. Apply the mixture onto your face avoiding the areas around eyes and mouth. Allow it to sink in for about 15 minutes. Wash your face with lukewarm water. This action loosens your face mask. Finally, rinse off the mask with cold water. Pat your face dry with a clean towel.

Benefits: Papaya is rich in beta-carotene, powerful enzymes, and phytochemicals. The secret beauty ingredient in papaya is papain that has skin lightening properties and reduces the visibility of blemishes and acne scars. Along with alpha hydroxyacids, papain acts as a gentle exfoliator that dissolves inactive protein and dead skin cells.

Papaya contains vitamins A and C, papain, alpha hydroxyl acids and potassium. Papain promotes skin regeneration; vitamin C boosts collagen production, vitamin A smoothens out aging skin. The potassium moisturizes your skin.

Cucumber has skin lightening properties and nourishes and moisturizes your skin.

Banana reduces wrinkles and promotes youthful, glowing skin.

Walnut and Milk Cream Pack

Things Needed

- 4-5 pieces Walnuts
- 1 Tbs milk cream

Method: Soak the nuts in water for one hour and mash them into a thick paste. Add the milk cream and mix well. Clean your face and neck and apply the walnut, dairy cream mask. Massage your face in soft circular motions for five minutes. Leave the mask for 20 minutes and wash off with water.

Benefits: Walnuts are powerhouses of omega 3 fatty acids. These fatty acids help to lock in moisture and nutrients into the skin making it plump and glowing. The omega 3 fats reduce the skin inflammation and protect your skin against harmful UV rays. The vitamin E present in walnuts accelerates skin healing and makes your skin smooth and glowing.

Milk removes oil based impurities with the help of enzyme lipase, protein based impurities with the aid of protease and dead skin cells with the support of the lactic acid. It lightens your skin by shedding off pigmented skin cells. Milk cream significantly reduces tan, dark spots, and dark patches.

Mint Face Mask

Ingredients

- Mint leaves 200 grams (paste)
- Cucumber 1 (paste)
- Green tea 1 cup
- Yogurt- 3 tablespoons
- Lemon 1 (juice)

Method: In a bowl add the mint leaves paste, cucumber paste, and yogurt. Mix the ingredients gently.Otherwise, you can blend all the three together in a blender.Now add the lemon juice and mix well. Store in a cool place for 20 minutes.

Wash your face with cold running water. Clean your face with a face wash and pat dry. Apply a thin layer of the mint pack onto your face gently. Allow it to dry. When the maskgets dried, apply another fresh coat and leave it for 20 minutes. Try to peel the mask once it is dry. Then wash your face with warm green tea. Don't wipe the tea. Allow it to dry on your skin. After 20 minutes rinse your face with ordinary water. For best results use this face pack twice a month.

Benefits: Mint juice is an excellent skin cleanser. It soothes your skin and is a good way to reduce pimples. Mint can relieve some of the symptoms of acne. Mint leaves tighten and cleanse your skin pores thus leaving you with oil free skin tone. Mint juice fights dark circles and puffiness of eyes. Green tea improves your skin complexion. A 2003 study by the Medical College of Georgia says that green tea aids in skin rejuvenation. Green tea flushes out toxins, reduces inflammation, heals blemishes and scars and even improves the elasticity of your skin.

Rose Face Mask

Ingredients

- 10 fresh rose petals
- 3 Tbs thick yogurt
- 2 Tbs of dried orange peel powder or ½ cup orange peels

Method: Add the fresh rose petals, yogurt, and orange peels or orange peel powder in your blender. Blend it to form semi smooth paste. Apply this face pack onto your face and neck. Leave the face pack for about 20 minutes and then wash it off using cold water.

Benefits: Rose petals contain cleansing and antibacterial properties. It is the best remedy to treat acne and acne prone skin. Rose provides a high amount of vitamin C which boosts your collagen production and plumps up your skin volume that naturally makes your skin radiant.

The natural oils present in rose help to store up moisture and hydrate your skin. The pleasant fragrance of the rose petals relaxes calms and soothes your stressed mind. As a natural astringent, rose restores your glowing complexion.

The peels remove dust and pollutants from pores and removes tan. Orange peels work as a natural bleach and lighten dark blotches. If you use them regularly, it completely removes them. They help lighten suntan and deflect the harmful UV rays.

Blackberry Saffron Face Mask

Things Needed

- ¼ cup Blackberries
- 1 Tbsp Aloe Gel
- A few strands of saffron

Method: Add the blackberries, saffron strands, and aloe gel into your blender. Blend to form a smooth paste. Transfer the contents to a glass bowl. Apply gently onto your face in circular motions.

Allow the mask to dry for 20-25 minutes and wash off with lukewarm water.

Benefits: Blackberries contain an abundance of antioxidants anthocyanocides and polyphenols which fight free radicals. The presence of vitamins A and C boosts your collagen production. Blackberries are composed of 85 percent of water which hydrates and moisturizes your skin. The vitamins A, C, and K in blackberries rejuvenate your facial skin and enhances your beauty.

Saffron is an excellent skin toning agent. It eliminates blackheads and unclogs the clogged pores. It is packed with A, C and B vitamins and possesses good skin lightening properties.

Aloe contains antibacterial and antioxidant properties. It reduces acne and lightens blemishes. It prevents wrinkles and acts as a natural moisturizer.

Carrot Face Pack

Ingredients

- ½ carrot
- ½ cup papaya pieces
- Egg white from one egg
- One tablespoon milk

Method: Put the carrot, papaya, egg white and milk into a blender. Blend it to form a smooth paste. Apply the carrot face mask onto your face in circular motions. Leave for 30 minutes and wash your face in the lukewarm water. Since you're using egg white using a gentle face wash will remove the odor.

Benefits: Carrots are rich in beta-carotene which gets converted to vitamin A in your body. It helps to repair the skin's tissue and protects against the sun's harsh rays. The vitamin A makes your skin color more attractive by imparting a healthy glow.

Adding more carrots to your daily diet will give a healthy dose of vitamin C that makes your skin firm and plump.

Egg white removes your facial hair. They have astringent properties that help shrink pores by tightening the skin. The nutrients in egg whites help to lift the sagging cheeks and crinkly skin around the eyes. Regular use of egg white masks reduces white heads while the protein in them heals and nourishes your skin.

Coconut Milk Face Pack

Ingredients

- 4 pieces Almonds
- 2 Tbsp freshly prepared coconut milk
- 1 tsp milk powder
- 1 tsp lime juice

Method: Soak the almonds overnight. Blend the almonds, coconut milk and lime juice in a blender. Mix in the milk powder. Clean your face and neck. Apply this mask allover your face and neck. Let the mask sit for 30 minutes then wash your face in the tepid water and gently pat dry.

Benefits: Coconut milk contains lauric acid, caprylic acid and capric acid which gives it antimicrobial and exceptional soothing qualities. Coconut milk is the best way to pamper your dehydrated skin. The proteins, vitamins, iron and calcium present in coconut milk nourishes your skin, improves skin elasticity thereby prevents and reduces sagging and wrinkling in your face. Coconut milk is rich in vitamin c that gives a healthy glow to your skin.

Almonds are rich in omega 3 fatty acids, proteins, magnesium and calcium. Almonds greatly enhance your complexion because it contains abundant amounts of vitamin E.

Vitamin E prevents cell damage and reinvigorates the cells, so your face looks fresh and glowing. The proteins present in almond milk soften and nourishes your skin. The omega 3 fatty acids present in almonds fight inflammation and keep your facial skin bright, young and beautiful.

Almond Oil & Banana Face Mask

This mask is effective for lightening skin tone. Banana is a powerhouse of vitamins B6 and C, so it helps to **improve the collagen production** that helps to maintain the elasticity and suppleness of the skin. Vitamin C aids in improving your complexion as well.

The benefits of almond oil for the skin are well known. Almonds are enriched with vitamins A, D, and E that act as beneficial **natural antioxidants for promoting skin health**. They also contain amazing anti-inflammatory properties, which help to soothe skin infections and allergies as well. Almonds may also help to lighten dark circles, improve circulation of blood throughout the skin, and fight the effects of harmful UV rays as well.

Ingredients

- 1 ripe banana
- 1 tsp. sweet almond oil

Directions

1. First, mash a banana well to create a smooth paste and then add the almond oil.
2. Mix well and apply this paste on your clean face.
3. Leave on for 20 minutes and wash well with warm water.

Cucumber & Tomato Face Mask

Tomatoes contain the antioxidant lycopene that acts as a great natural sunscreen and helps to **soothe the skin against sunburn**. In addition, its natural astringent agents help to lower the open pore's size and curb the skin's excessive oiliness. Moreover, it adds a natural glow to lifeless, dull skin.

Cucumber pulp and juice also act as a beneficial natural remedy for enhancing the complexion by **eliminating blemishes, pigmentation, and scars**. It is also a natural and effective remedy for lowering cellulite and lightening dark circles under the eyes.

Ingredients

- 1 small tomato
- ½ cucumber, peeled

Directions

1. Mash the tomato into a smooth paste.
2. Grate half a cucumber and mix the grated cucumber with the tomato paste.
3. Apply on your clean face and leave for 20 minutes before washing off with water.

Sandalwood & Orange Peel Face Mask

Sandalwood has been used for skin problems since ancient times. It also holds a vital place in Ayurvedic treatment.

Orange peels are filled with vitamin C and calcium. Vitamin C has the ability to **neutralize skin damage** caused by harmful free radicals as well as oxidative stress. In addition, it serves as a useful natural cure to **keep blackheads on the nose at bay**. Its natural bleaching qualities help fade dark patches and effectively improve skin tone. This face mask not only exfoliates the skin but also tones it.

Ingredients

- 1 Tbsp. orange peel powder
- 1 Tbsp. sandalwood powder

Directions

1. Add both powders to a small glass bowl, and mix in enough water to make a thick paste.
2. Apply to face and neck and massage gently for five minutes.
3. Let the mask set for 15 minutes before washing off with warm water.

Walnut & Milk Cream Face Mask

Milk cream functions as a natural moisturizer for excessively flaky and dry skin. It works as a great toner that enhances skin tone and adds an immediate healthy glow to your skin. Milk cream is also a great natural cure for bags and dark circles under the eyes.

Walnuts are full of antioxidants, B vitamins, and vitamin E. These nutrients help to **improve overall skin health** by counteracting skin damage caused due to oxidative stress and free radicals, reducing the aging process

Ingredients

- 4 to 5 organic walnuts
- 1 Tbsp. milk cream

Directions

1. Soak the walnuts in water for around 60 minutes; drain and mash well to create a thick paste.
2. Add the milk cream and mix well.
3. Apply this mixture on your clean neck and face and massage for 5 minutes in a soft circular motion.
4. Let sit for 20 minutes before washing off with water.

Papaya and Honey Face Mask

Ripe papaya contains the enzyme papain, which helps in skin renewal. In addition, vitamins A, C, and E, as well as antioxidants, help to moisturize the skin and protect it against infections. Papaya also helps to decrease skin aging signs such as age spots and freckles.

Ingredients

- ½ cup ripe papaya
- 1 tsp. honey

Directions

Mash the papaya to create a thick, smooth paste.

Add the honey and mix well.

Smooth onto the face and let rest for 20 minutes before washing off with water.

Lemon & Potato Pulp Face Mask

Lemon acts as a wonderful natural bleaching agent. It is often used in hair care routines and consists of lots of skin benefits such as eliminating dead skin cells and impurities.

Potato juice and pulp both are a traditional cure for lightening the skin, improving skin health, and removing blemishes. Potatoes are also a powerhouse of vitamin C, which helps to nourish the skin from within. It also functions as an effective natural cure for removing dark spots and hyperpigmentation. Last but not least, it improves skin tone and lightens dark circles around eyes.

Ingredients

- 1 small potato
- 1 lemon

Directions

Peel and grate the potato into a smooth pulp.

Extract the juice of a lemon and add to the pulp.

Mix well and apply this mask on your clean face for 20 minutes before washing off.

Yogurt & Oatmeal Face Mask

This skin whitening face mask serves as an effective natural cure for **fading age spots, suntan, and pigmentation** as well. Oatmeal is extremely useful for exfoliating the skin, removing impurities and dead cells, and enhancing the fairness of skin.

Unflavored yogurt has high levels of alpha hydroxy acid and lactic acid that help to moisturize and exfoliate the skin. As a result, it makes the skin smooth and glowing as well. Its mild bleaching properties also help to correct age spots and skin discoloration.

Yogurt has the capacity to prevent the breakout of pimples and acne.

Ingredients

- 2 Tbsp. yogurt
- 1 Tbsp. oats

Directions

1. In a glass bowl, whisk the oats into the yogurt.
2. Mix well and apply this combination on your face, arms, and neck; massaging for five minutes using a circular motion.
3. Let rest for 20 minutes and wash off thoroughly using water.

Milk & Honey Face Mask

Honey is nature's elixir for all problems of the skin. Being an awesome **natural antibacterial agent**, honey acts as an excellent natural remedy for pimples and acne. It helps to moisturize excessively dry skin and add a natural glow to the skin as well. Raw milk, on the other hand, is a wonderful skin cleanser that **helps to improve complexion**.

Ingredients

- 1 Tbsp. honey
- 1 Tbsp. raw milk

Directions

Mix the honey and raw milk in a glass bowl. Apply to your clean face and massage for two minutes in a soft, circular motion. Let the mask rest for 20 minutes before washing off with water.

Honey and Milk glowing face mask

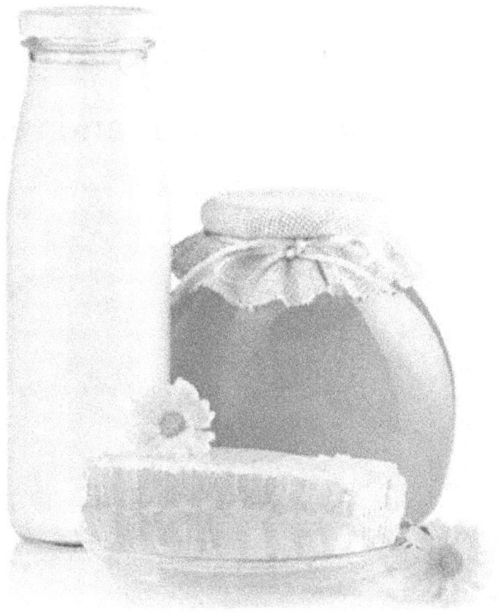

Ingredients

Honey-1 Tablespoon Raw Milk-1 Tablespoon

Directions

Mix the ingredients in a glass bowl and apply on clean face, massage for 2 minutes in soft, circular motion, leave on for 15 to 20 minutes and wash off thoroughly with water.

Potato Pulp and Lemon Pack

Potato juice and pulp are an age-old home remedy for skin lightening, removing blemishes and improving skin health and is a nourishing homemade facial for oily skin.

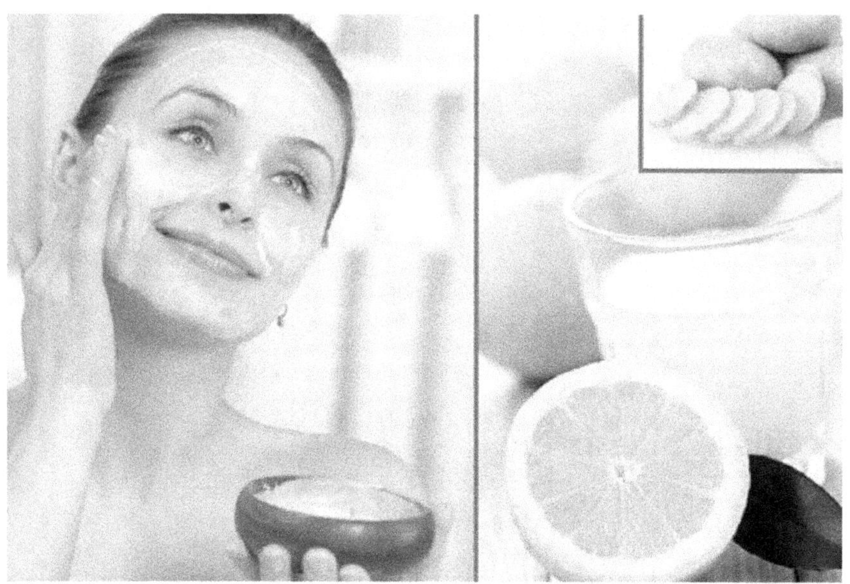

Ingredients

- Potato 1
- Small Lemon 1

Directions

Peel and grate the potato to turn it into smooth pulp, squeeze out the juice of one lemon and add it to the pulp, mix well and apply on clean face, let it stay for 20 minutes and wash off with water.

Yogurt and Oats Pack

This is the best skin whitening face pack that acts as an effective natural remedy for removing suntan, age spots and pigmentation. The benefits of oatmeal for health are well known, but it is also extremely beneficial for exfoliating the skin as well to remove dead cells and impurities and improving the fairness of skin.

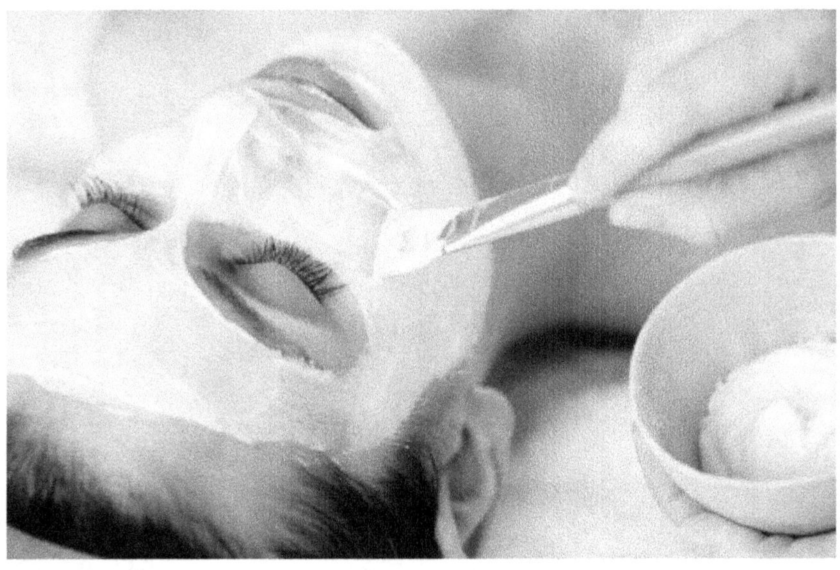

Ingredients

- Yogurt 2 tablespoons
- Oats 1 Tablespoon

Directions

Whisk the yogurt in a glass bowl and add the oats to it, mix well and apply on face, neck and arms, massage using soft motion on face, neck and arms for 5 minutes, leave it on for 20 minutes and wash off thoroughly with water.

Banana and Almond Oil Pack

One of the easiest and most cost effective homemade face packs for lightening skin tone can be made from ripe bananas and almond oil. It is the best deep nourishing moisturizer for dry skin that also helps in lightening dark circles, protects the skin against the harmful UV rays of the sun and improves blood circulation throughout the skin.

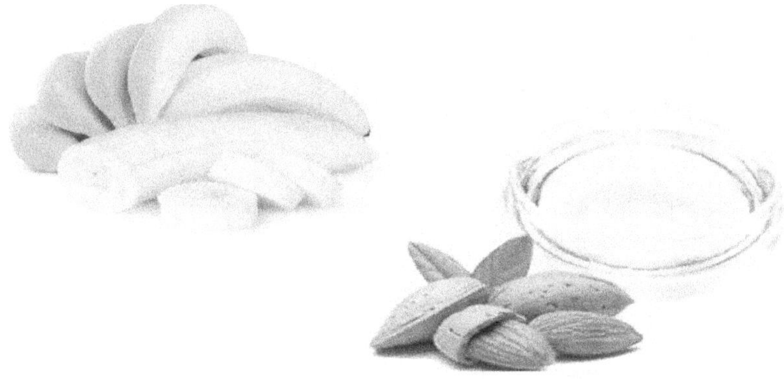

Ingredients

- Ripe Banana 1
- Sweet Almond Oil 1 Tea Spoon

Directions

Mash the banana, well to form a smooth paste, add the almond oil to it, mix well and apply on clean face, let it stay for 20 minutes and wash off well with water.

Orange Peel and Sandalwood Pack

This is the most effective face pack for skin whitening that also exfoliates and tones the skin at the same time.

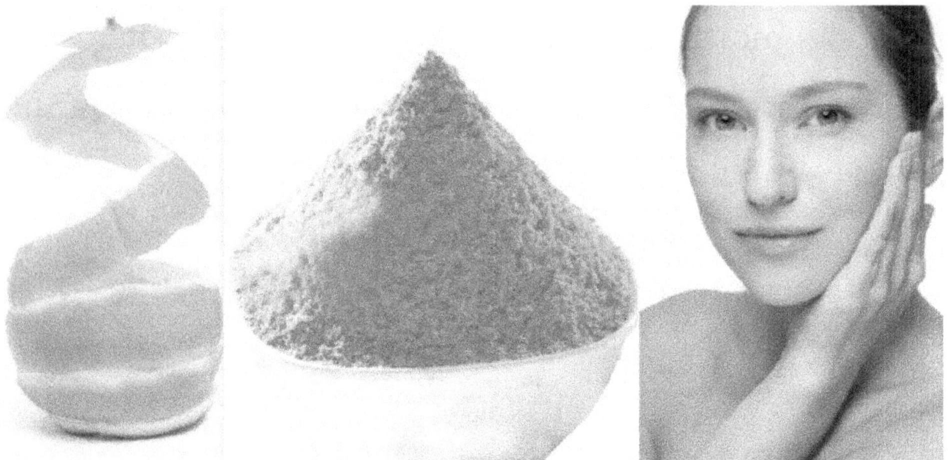

Ingredients

- Orange Peel Powder 1 Tablespoon
- Sandalwood Powder 1 Tablespoon

Directions

Mix orange peel powder and sandalwood powder in a glass bowl and add some water to it to have a thick consistency, apply it on clean face and neck, massage for 5 minutes, leave it on for 15 minutes and wash off with water.

Turmeric and Gram Flour Pack

The health benefits of turmeric are well known. Turmeric is a widely used kitchen spice in India and it holds a very important place in auspicious Hindu ceremonies such as marriages where turmeric or "Haldi" paste in applied on the bride and bridegroom's face and body. It works as an amazing natural remedy for nourishing dry skin and removing impurities and dead cells from the skin.

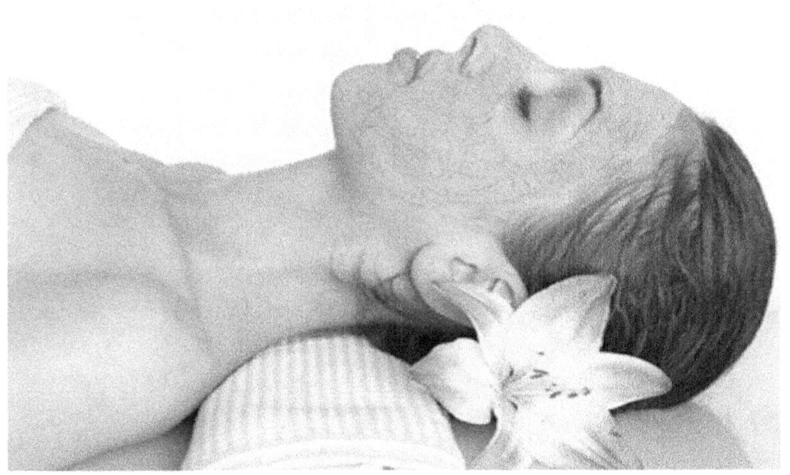

Ingredients
- Turmeric Paste 1 Teaspoon
- Gram Flour 1 Tablespoon

Directions
Mix the turmeric paste and gram flour in a glass bowl and add 1 tablespoon of milk to it, blend well and apply on clean face, let it stay for 15 minutes and wash off well with water.

Tomato and Cucumber Skin glowing Pack

Tomatoes can be used effectively in a fairness face pack to enhance the skin tone naturally. The antioxidant lycopene present in tomatoes acts as a natural sunscreen and soothes the skin against sunburn. It helps in adding a natural glow to dull, lifeless skin.

Cucumber juice and pulp act as an effective natural remedy for improving the complexion by removing pigmentation, blemishes and scars. It functions like a natural remedy for reducing cellulite and also works in lightening dark circles around eyes.

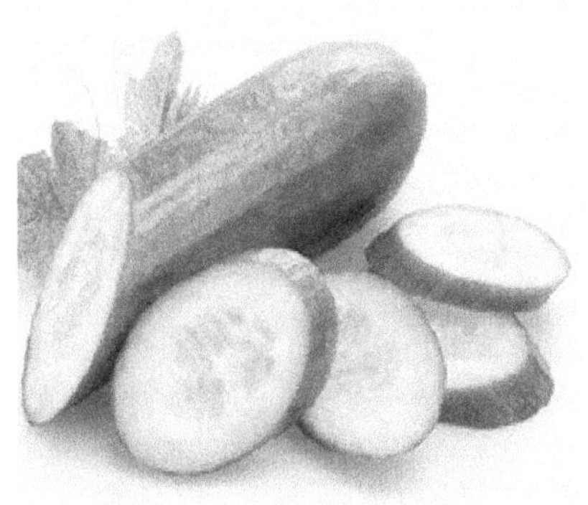 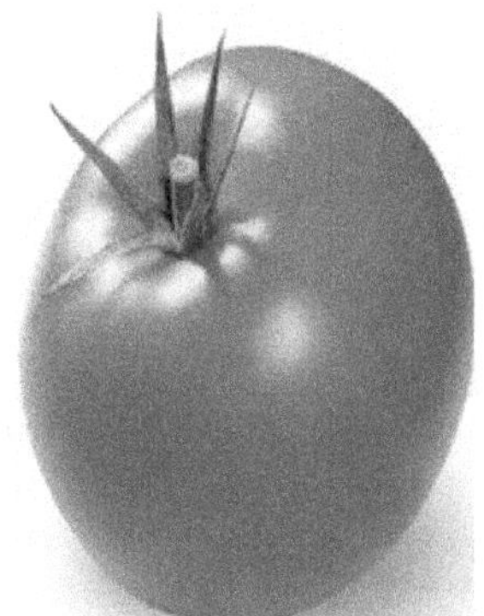

Ingredients

- Tomato - 1
- Small Cucumber - 1/2 Peeled

Directions

Mash the tomato to form a smooth paste and grate ½ cucumber and mix it with the tomato paste. Apply the paste on clean face and let it stay for 20 minutes, wash off with water.

Walnut and Milk Cream Pack

Walnuts are loaded with antioxidants, vitamin E and B vitamins that help in improving overall skin health by neutralizing skin damage caused by free radicals and oxidative stress and slowing the process of aging. Milk cream is the best natural moisturizer for excessive dry and flaky skin. It also acts as a soothing skin toner that helps in improving skin tone and adding an instant healthy glow to the skin.

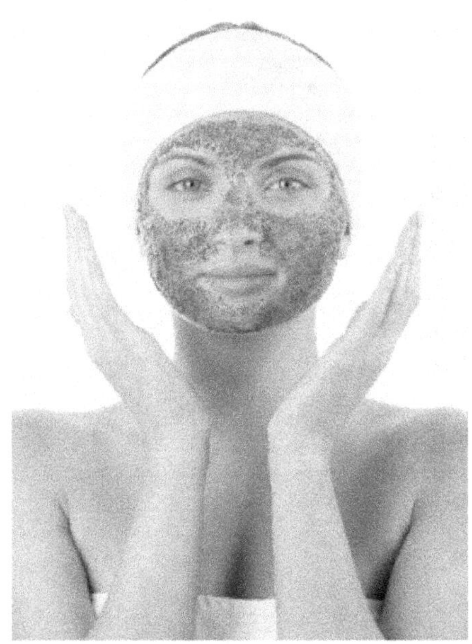

Ingredients

Walnuts - 4 to 5

Milk Cream-1 Tablespoon

Directions

Soak the walnuts in water for 1 hour and mash them into a thick paste, add the milk cream to it and mix well. Apply this mixture on clean face and neck and massage in soft circular motion for 5 minutes, leave it on for 20 minutes and wash off with water.

Strawberry and Milk Skin Whitening Pack

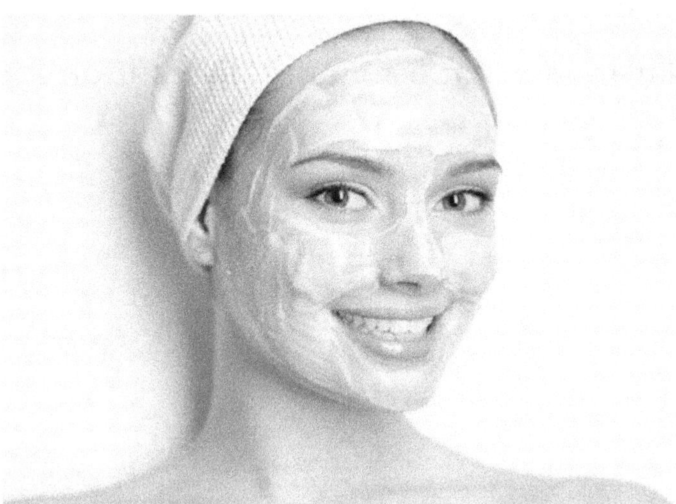

Ingredients

- Ripe Strawberries-2
- Raw Milk-1 tablespoon

Directions

Mash the ripe strawberries to form a smooth paste, add raw milk to it and mix well. Apply this mixture on clean face and let it stay for 20 minutes, wash off with water.

www.ingramcontent.com/pod-product-compliance
Lightning Source LLC
Chambersburg PA
CBHW081809250726
48653CB00010B/3860